CHILDHOOD ASTHMA

A SELF-MANAGEMENT PROGRAM FOR THE ENTIRE FAMILY

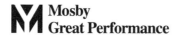

Mosby
Great Performance

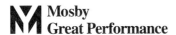

Developmental Editor: Stephanie Slon
Assistant Editor: Katherine Eklund
Production Manager: Christine Jennings
Production Coordinator: Jeremy Wells
Designer: Kirk Peeler
Cover Illustration: Nancy Olson
Illustrations: Lori Vascalles

First Edition

Special thanks to clinical consultants:

James M. Dover, M.D.
Allergy Department Chairperson
Thomas-Davis Medical Centers

David Gluck, M.D.
Fellow, American College of Preventive Medicine

Spenser Roberts, M.S.
Health Educator for Intergroup Health Care Corporation
Director—Asthma Education Program

James W. Villaveces, M.D., A.B.A.I.
Fellow, American Academy of Allergy-Immunology
Fellow, American College of Allergy-Immunology

The material in this publication is for general information only and is not intended to provide specific advice or recommendations for any individual. Your physician or other health professional must be consulted for advice with regard to your individual situation.

ISBN 0-8151-9595-8 / 26513

Printed on recycled paper.

FOREWORD

Living well with any chronic condition requires a unique combination of skills. First, it involves learning as much as you can about your problem—everything from what's happening in your body to how different medications work. Next, it takes time and effort to form a solid partnership with members of your health care team. This includes the doctors, nurses, pharmacists, educators, and therapists who will be working with you. Being an active partner in health care means that you prepare for your visits, you actively seek answers to questions, and you completely understand treatment recommendations.

Self-management also requires that you learn how to track and monitor your condition. You recognize warning signs that signal the need to see your doctor and you learn what problems can be handled yourself.

These are important skills in caring for any medical problem. There's something else that determines much of how you look and feel. It's the lifestyle choices you make every day in nutrition, appropriate physical activity and stress-management. These changes start with a willingness to change, a can-do attitude, and a long-range perspective.

In the pages ahead, you'll find helpful information in all of these areas.

For almost 100 years, the Mosby company has provided your doctors, nurses, and allied health professionals with the latest information and advances in medicine. We're proud now to bring these same quality resources to help you gain the necessary knowledge, skills, and support for the best of health.

Mark J. Tager, m.o.

Mark J. Tager, M.D.
President, Mosby-Great Performance, Inc.

TABLE OF CONTENTS

INTRODUCTION

You **Can** Help Your Child

There's nothing more frightening than seeing your child struggle to breathe. Hundreds of thousands of parents have spent anxious hours in hospital emergency rooms, hoping and praying that their child would recover from the latest asthma episode. If your child has asthma, you're not alone. The American Lung Association estimates that more than 4 million children in the United States have asthma. Other experts suggest the number is even higher, because thousands of children have "hidden" asthma that goes undiagnosed or misdiagnosed. Asthma is one of the most common chronic illnesses among children under 18 and the number one cause of childhood hospitalizations. It's a major cause of school absenteeism, causing the average child with asthma to miss 12 days of school every year. It's a serious disease that, left uncontrolled and untreated, can even lead to death.

Like many parents of children with asthma, the disease probably makes you feel helpless and guilty. You may wonder if there isn't something you can do to prevent your child from having another frightening asthma episode. The good news is that there is. In recent years, health care experts have expanded our understanding of what asthma is. While they don't have a cure for this chronic lung disease, new drugs and devices are better able to prevent asthma symptoms and to control them when they do occur. Doctors rely more heavily than ever on parents and children to learn self-management techniques like avoiding asthma "triggers" and responding promptly to the early warning signs of asthma.

Asthma doesn't have to control your family's life. Instead of waiting anxiously for the next asthma flare-up, you can take charge and learn to control your child's asthma. By working closely with your doctor and other health care providers, you and your child can lead a normal life without restrictions because of asthma. With proper asthma management, your child can expect to have normal (or near normal) lung function, be able to participate in the same activities as other children, prevent and/or minimize asthma symptoms, and eliminate or decrease the incidence of asthma episodes.

It's important for all parents to take an active role in the health care of their children. It's even more important when your child has asthma. To help your child effectively manage his or her asthma, you need to:

Continue to learn all you can about asthma and teach your child about it. Researchers are learning more all the time about the disease and more effective ways to treat it. Even if you've been dealing with your child's asthma for some time now, you need to continue to learn. This book is a great first step.

Teach your child self-management techniques and help your child take charge of managing his or her asthma. There are plenty of things you can do to help your child manage his or her asthma. These include ensuring your child takes the proper medication at the right time, helping your child identify and avoid asthma "triggers," teaching your child to recognize and respond promptly to early warning signs of a flare-up, and encouraging your child to stay physically active.

Become an active and involved member of your child's health care team. You, your child, your doctor, nurse, pharmacist, and other health care providers must all work together to manage your child's asthma.

Coordinate your child's asthma care with school personnel and other care providers. It's up to you to ensure that teachers, coaches, school nurses, and other care providers are informed and able to respond if your child needs help with his or her asthma symptoms.

You'll find the commitment and effort put into controlling your child's asthma well worth it. You'll be teaching your child how to manage the condition as he or she grows up. And you'll have peace of mind knowing you've done all you can to help your child have a healthy, active life.

Understanding Your Child's Asthma

The first step in taking control of your child's asthma is learning all you can about it. This section will help you understand what asthma is, what causes it, its signs and symptoms, and how doctors diagnose it.

Common Myths About Asthma

Before we get into exactly what asthma is, let's first look at some of the most common myths about asthma.

"Only children get asthma." It's true that many people are diagnosed with asthma in childhood. However, adults can develop asthma too.

"Asthma is a disease children outgrow." Children's asthma may improve after a child reaches about age 10. However, the improvement isn't because the child has "outgrown" the disease, but because the diameter of the child's airways has increased as he or she has grown. The airways remain sensitive to the conditions that can bring on asthma flare-ups.

"Asthma is contagious." Your child didn't "catch" asthma, and he or she can't "give" it to anyone else.

"Overprotective or negligent parenting can cause a child to get asthma." Asthma is entirely a lung problem and is unrelated to your parenting skills. Helping your child understand and accept his or her illness, however, can have a dramatic impact on your child's ability to control his or her asthma.

"Asthma flare-ups are uncomfortable and inconvenient, but they aren't really dangerous." Asthma can be serious and even fatal if not properly treated. The belief that no one dies from asthma is false. Because the airways of infants are less developed, babies with asthma

are especially at risk for serious flare-ups. Your commitment to helping your child manage his or her asthma can help prevent serious episodes and help your child lead a healthy, normal life.

"It's my fault my child is asthmatic." It's no more a parent's "fault" his or her child has asthma than it is his or her "fault" the child has brown eyes or red hair. The tendency to get asthma runs in families. If one parent has asthma, one in four children are likely to have it. If both parents have asthma, half of all children in the family are likely to develop it at some age. A child does not inherit the age at which he or she will develop the disease, what will trigger it, or how severe it will be—only the tendency to develop it.

As a parent, you are responsible if you expose your child to cigarette smoke in the house or other environmental irritants that can bring on an asthma episode. Children growing up in a home with parents who smoke have four times the respiratory problems of other children.

"Asthma leads to emphysema and other lung diseases." Asthma isn't related to emphysema or other lung problems.

"Asthma is progressive." Your child's asthma may get worse or it may get better. Unlike other airway diseases such as cystic fibrosis or emphysema, asthma doesn't automatically get progressively worse.

"Children who have asthma have psychological problems that cause their condition." Asthma is a lung problem, not a psychological disease. Children who have asthma are no more prone to major psychological problems than other children. However, parents must be aware that any chronic disease such as asthma can cause children a wide range of feelings like anger, resentment, and depression. With your help and support, your child can work through these emotions and live a full and active life.

What Is Asthma?

Now that you know what asthma isn't, let's find out what it is. Asthma is a long-term (chronic) disease of the lungs that causes tiny airways of the lungs, called *bronchioles*, to become inflamed (swollen) and narrowed or blocked, making it difficult to breathe. The airway inflammation causes the lining of the airways to leak extra mucus, making it even harder to breathe. Another aspect of asthma is lung hyperactivity, brought on by the inflammation. The lung reacts now to cold air, smoke and odors. When a child has asthma, he or she may experience shortness of breath, wheezing, coughing, and chest tightness. Or the child may be less active, have frequent bouts of bronchitis, and only cough chronically at night. Your child may experience all or only some of these symptoms. In some children, for example, coughing is their only asthma symptom.

If you could see inside your child's lungs, they would look like an upside down tree. The windpipe *(trachea)* is the tree's trunk. The two main air pipes *(bronchi)* are the tree's main branches off the trunk. One bronchial tube branches into each lung. These bronchi become the bronchial tree's "limbs," smaller airways called *bronchioles*. At the ends of each of these small airways are tiny air sacs *(alveoli)*, the tree's "leaves." These spongy air sacs receive fresh oxygen and exchange it for the waste product carbon dioxide.

When your child breathes, air comes in through the nose and mouth, where it is warmed and moistened so it doesn't damage the delicate lining of the airways. Then it passes through the windpipe and into the lungs through the two large bronchi. Finally, the air moves into the small air tubes and into the air sacs, where oxygen is transferred into the blood and carbon dioxide is moved into the sacs to be exhaled.

The airways have a delicate lining *(mucosa)* that is coated with a thin layer of mucus. This sticky mucus is important in keeping the airways clean and free of debris. The mucus traps foreign particles. With the help of the tiny finger-like projections *(cilia)* in the airways the mucus and particles are moved toward the mouth and nose where they are coughed or sneezed out or swallowed.

Tiny blood vessels that surround the airways keep harmful materials, such as bacteria and viruses, from doing damage by releasing substances that protect them. These protective cells, antibodies, and special proteins cause airway swelling. Muscles that surround the airways contract, and help trap, destroy, and remove these harmful foreign materials.

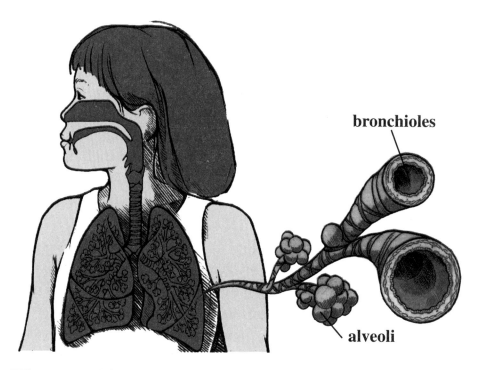

bronchioles

alveoli

When your child has asthma, the muscle contraction, mucosal swelling (inflammation), and mucus formation that normally protect the airways go haywire. Instead of reacting to only harmful foreign substances, the airways become supersensitive or "twitchy." They react to normally harmless substances and physical conditions such as pollen, animal dander, exercise, or cold air with muscle tightening (bronchospasm), swelling of the lining, and extra mucus production.

What Happens During an Asthma Flare-up?

When your child's coughing, wheezing, shortness of breath, and chest tightening become progressively worse, doctors call it an "asthma episode," "asthma flare," or "asthma flare-up." These episodes can be mild and short-lived, or quite severe and last for hours or even days and require hospitalization. They can occur once in a lifetime or every day.

During an asthma episode, several things happen:

1. The smooth muscles that surround the airways tighten (bronchospasm), causing the airways to narrow.

2. The lining of the airways swell, blocking the airways even more.

3. The mucus-producing glands in the airways produce excessive amounts of thick, sticky mucus that can block airways.

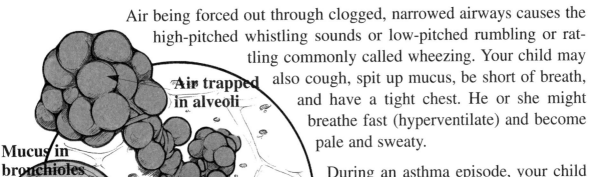

Air being forced out through clogged, narrowed airways causes the high-pitched whistling sounds or low-pitched rumbling or rattling commonly called wheezing. Your child may also cough, spit up mucus, be short of breath, and have a tight chest. He or she might breathe fast (hyperventilate) and become pale and sweaty.

Air trapped in alveoli

Mucus in bronchioles

Swelling and contracted muscles

During an asthma episode, your child may feel like he or she can't breathe in enough air. Actually, the child can't breathe *out* enough air. Stale, oxygen-poor air becomes trapped behind the tiny airways, leaving less room for fresh air to be inhaled. If the asthma episode is severe, your child's blood may become low in oxygen (hypoxemia).

Asthma flares can occur at any time. However, they are more common during the nighttime or early morning hours. Health care experts aren't sure why children (and adults) have more asthma attacks at night. Some speculate that breathing cooler night air irritates the airways and triggers symptoms. Other researchers suggest that the hormonal shifts (lower levels of adrenaline and cortisone, and higher levels of histamines) that occur at night may be a factor.

What Causes Asthma?

Researchers aren't sure why some children develop these super-sensitive airways while others don't. Asthma appears to run in families, but it can skip generations. Some children carry the predisposition to asthma and never develop symptoms. Others are not so lucky.

While doctors understand some of what happens during an asthma episode, they're not sure what causes it. One theory suggests that children who have asthma produce too much of the antibody immunoglobulin E (IgE), a special protective antibody that reacts to everyday substances in the environment. Children whose bodies produce a lot of IgE may develop allergies, hayfever, or asthma.

Other researchers believe asthma is caused by a defect in the lung cells' beta receptors. These so-called "defective" beta receptors, say scientists, cause the nervous system to overreact and cause bronchospasms. No one knows exactly why some children have defective beta receptors. Some suggest the damage may be genetic, while others say viral infections may cause the problem.

Recently, researchers have discovered that the airways of those with asthma remain inflamed, even after more obvious asthma symptoms have subsided. In fact, it may take as long as seven days for the lungs to recover completely after the wheezing stops. Experts believe this long-term irritation may be a key cause of asthma symptoms, and this knowledge has substantially changed how they treat asthma. However, no one is sure exactly what causes this chronic airway inflammation. It may be that when irritants come in contact with specialized cells in the airway lining, these cells leak chemicals such as histamine and prostaglandins. These, in turn, stimulate the muscle contraction, swelling, and increased mucus production.

What Role Do Allergies Play?

If your child has asthma it's likely he or she also has allergies and that you or others in your family suffer from allergies too. The majority (75 to 85 percent) of children with asthma have allergies. Substances outside the body such as dust, pollen, or food cause the body to release chemicals like histamine, which cause the asthma symptoms.

Your child may be allergic to only a few substances (allergens) or to many. Some children are allergic only to specific plants or to seasonal pollens. Studies of children with asthma suggest that the more substances your child is allergic to, the more severe his or her asthma is likely to be.

Allergens can cause your child to have an **immediate** or a **delayed** allergic reaction. In an **immediate response**, the child exposed to an asthma trigger like grass pollen may cough, wheeze, and have chest tightness and difficulty breathing within five to ten minutes of exposure. Symptoms from an immediate allergic reaction are likely to last from $1^1/_2$ to 2 hours. Common immediate response triggers include exercise, cold air, histamine, emotional stress, and irritants like cigarette smoke and air pollution.

A **delayed reaction** can come several hours after exposure to the offensive substance. Doctors say delayed allergic reactions are likely due to airway inflammation and the resulting damage to cells in the lining of the airways. The inflammation causes the airways to become hyper-responsive and this sensitivity may last for several weeks, even after only one exposure to the asthma trigger.

Some children with asthma have both immediate and delayed reactions to allergens. This **dual response** occurs because, after the initial symptoms stop, the airways may be left inflamed and super-sensitive. The second asthma episode can begin hours or even days after the first episode and is usually more severe than the immediate response.

Is My Child's Asthma Triggered by Allergies?

You may already suspect that your child has allergies that trigger his or her asthma. Maybe you've noticed that your child develops asthma symptoms during certain months in spring or summer. Or perhaps your child's symptoms are triggered when he or she is in a dusty environment or after he or she has handled the family pet. Your doctor can conduct skin tests to pinpoint specific allergies, or you may be referred to an allergist who will do the skin tests.

All of the allergens listed below are small and light enough to be carried on the wind for long periods of time. For some children, even a brief exposure to very small amounts of the allergens will produce asthma symptoms when the allergens are inhaled deeply into the lungs.

Common Asthma-Triggering Allergens

- Pollens (grasses, trees, ragweed).

- Mold spores (greenhouses, damp basements).

- Animal dander/feathers (rabbits, cats, dogs, birds, hamsters, gerbils, chickens, horses, guinea pigs, mice).

- Dust mites (rugs, draperies, bedding, dirty air and furnace filters).

Identifying Possible Triggers of Asthma

Use the following checklist, adapted from the National Institutes of Health.

❏ *Is your child's asthma worse in certain months? If so, does your child have asthma symptoms as well as sneezing, itching, runny and/or stuffed-up nose?*

Your child may be allergic to pollens and outdoor molds.

❏ *Do your child's symptoms appear when he or she visits where there are indoor pets?*

Your child may be allergic to animal dander, saliva, and urine.

❏ *If you have pets in your home, do your child's symptoms improve when he or she is away from home for a week or longer? Do the child's symptoms return or get worse the first 24 hours after returning home?*

Your child may be allergic to animal dander and saliva.

❏ *Do your child's eyes become red after handing pets? If the pet licks the child, does it produce red, itchy welts?*

Your child may be allergic to animal dander.

❏ *Does your child experience asthma symptoms when he or she is in a room where the carpets are being vacuumed?*

Your child may be allergic to dust mites or animal dander.

❏ *Does your child develop symptoms when he or she makes the bed?*
Your child may be allergic to dust mites.

❏ *Does your child experience symptoms when around hay or in a barn or stable?*

Your child may be allergic to molds.

❏ *Do symptoms develop when your child goes into a greenhouse, damp basement, or vacation cottage that has been closed up for some time?*

Your child may be allergic to molds.

Food allergies can also trigger asthma symptoms. True food allergies are more common in infants and children than in adults. They are often found in children with eczema, an allergic skin disorder that usually begins in infancy. Fortunately, four out of five of these asthma-eczema infants grow out of these conditions as older children.

Experts estimate that about five percent of children with asthma have food allergies. In a few children (less than one in 100), foods or food additives or preservatives like sulfites and sulfur dioxide, among others, can produce a significant allergic reaction. In others, they may produce a low-grade reaction. However, daily exposure to these foods or food substances may result in a gradual worsening of the child's asthma.

Common Food Allergy Triggers in Children

- Citrus fruits
- Fish
- Eggs
- Peanut butter
- Cow's milk and milk products
- Soy
- Wheat
- Fish
- Nuts
- Additives—for example, monosodium glutamate (MSG), sulfites, sulfur dioxide, Tartrazine, yellow dye No. 5

What Else Can Trigger My Child's Asthma?

In addition to food and environmental allergens like pollens, molds, dust mites, animal dander, and food, your child's asthma may be triggered by:

Irritants. Our modern air is full of airway irritants such as tobacco smoke (cigarettes, pipes, cigars), air pollution (car exhaust, industrial smog, smoke from burning fossil fuels), strong odors, aerosol sprays, and paint fumes. Even common household products like perfume, hair spray, cleaning fluids, chlorine bleach, and room deodorizers are known bronchial irritants. These substances can irritate your child's lungs and upper airways and cause the same cough, wheeze, runny-nose, watery-eyes reactions that allergens do.

Cigarette smoke is one of the more common asthma triggers for children. It contains dozens of irritating chemicals, including nicotine, carbon monoxide, pesticides, and insecticides. Whether the smoke is direct or secondary smoke—smoke from other people's cigarettes—this irritant can be especially harmful to children with asthma. In fact, studies now show direct correlations between parents' smoking and the frequency of children's asthma attacks. HEPA air filters can help clear the bedroom air of particulates and smoke.

Upper Respiratory Infections. Asthma in infants and young children is commonly triggered by infections like colds, flu, bronchitis, tonsillitis, sinusitis, and sore throat. Infants are especially vulnerable to respiratory syncytial virus (RSV), an infection that causes high fever and wheezing. Infections are so common among children with asthma, some researchers have found that as many as four in ten hospitalizations for childhood asthma are caused by common cold viruses. New guidelines suggest that children who get asthma flare-ups every time they get a cold may be treated with anti-inflammatory medicines at the first sign of the cold, before the asthma occurs.

As a parent of a child with asthma, you may feel your child has a cold all the time. Many children with asthma (or sinusitis, hayfever or viral infections) have a constantly itchy nose. Since colds are often transmitted by hand-to-mouth contact, kids who continually rub their noses (dubbed the "allergic salute") easily transfer viruses they pick up on their hands to their mouths.

Parents may be surprised if their child's doctor doesn't offer antibiotics for an infection. The truth is, many childhood infections are caused by viruses rather than bacteria. Antibiotics aren't effective against viruses. The doctor will only use antibiotics if he or she believes the child has an infection caused by bacteria, such as sinusitis or bronchitis. The buildup of mucus in the sinuses and lungs provides an excellent breeding ground for bacteria.

Sinusitis. Chronic childhood sinusitis (infection of the sinuses) can be a very potent asthma trigger for some children. At one time, researchers believed children had undeveloped sinuses and didn't get sinusitis. Now they know that even newborn infants can develop sinus infections.

Unfortunately, childhood sinusitis can be resistant to treatment. The standard 10-day antibiotic treatment may not be effective for your child's chronic sinusitis. He or she may require a longer (three to six weeks) course of antibiotics. Your doctor may also wish to order x-rays or a specialized local CT scan of the sinuses if infections are chronically recurrent.

Exercise. There's also a special category of asthma, **exercise-induced asthma or EIA** (also called exercise-induced bronchospasm or EIB), that's very common in children. During exercise, the bronchial tubes of an exercise-sensitive child tighten (constrict) rather than open up (dilate). Often six to eight minutes into physical activity, the child begins to wheeze, cough, feel short of breath, have chest pain or tightness, or feel tired. For other children, symptoms begin five to ten minutes after stopping exercise. Sometimes the asthma reaction is delayed and symptoms don't begin for several hours after physical activity.

Experts aren't sure why some children's bronchial tubes tighten during exercise. Most suspect it has something to do with a defect in the way inhaled air is warmed and moistened (humidified). In a child who doesn't have asthma, inhaled air arrives in the lungs moist and warmed to body temperature. However, in a child with asthma, the air arrives in the lungs cool and dry, causing a severe reaction in the bronchial tree.

Weather. A number of weather conditions can trigger asthma in children. Breathing cold air is a known asthma trigger. Climate changes can stimulate asthma too. High humidity and light rainfall can increase mold allergen levels in the air.

Sleeping (Nocturnal Asthma). Many children are bothered by night-time episodes of asthma. While your child sleeps, his or her airways may become narrow and collect mucus.

Emotions. An asthma factor for many children is emotion. It is commonly believed that children who have asthma have psychological problems. There's no evidence to support this myth. Asthma isn't "all in your child's head," it's "all in his or her lungs." Sometimes emotional stresses that cause your child to breathe rapidly, such as crying or laughing, can trigger an asthma attack. However, it's the rapid breathing that's the trigger rather than the emotions themselves.

Sometimes anger, frustration, anxiety and other strong emotions can trigger asthma. However, most asthma experts believe the asthma condition already existed and the emotion simply triggered a reaction. During an asthma attack, emotions like fear, anxiety, and panic can cause the child to breathe rapidly (hyperventilate) and make the episode worse.

Stress. Any emotional or physical stress, such as hunger, cold air, or even lack of rest, can contribute to asthma.

How Can I Tell If My Child Has Asthma?

Only your doctor can make an accurate asthma diagnosis. Unfortunately, asthma in children is frequently misdiagnosed. Often young children with asthma only wheeze when they have a respiratory infection and doctors may dismiss their symptoms as bronchitis or pneumonia. Also, a number of childhood illnesses such as croup, bronchitis, and cystic fibrosis have symptoms that can be confused with asthma. Infants can develop a viral infection of the bronchial tubes (broncholitis) caused by a potent virus called the respiratory syncytial virus (RSV). This respiratory infection causes high fever and a severe wheezing that doesn't respond to anti-wheezing medications. Young children often inhale foreign objects like beans or other small objects that lodge in the windpipe and cause wheezing similar to asthma, which can make an accurate diagnosis difficult. Another type of asthma is called cough-variant asthma, in which the child coughs instead of wheezing. This coughing can sometimes be misleading in diagnosis.

No one diagnostic test or set of tests is needed for every child. The doctor will order the tests he or she feels are needed to make an accurate diagnosis. Your child's diagnosis of asthma will likely be based on findings from:

- Your child's symptoms and medical history.

- The physical exam.

- Breathing (lung function) tests.

- Chest x-ray.

- Laboratory tests, including blood work.

- Skin tests for allergies.

- Sinus x-ray or mini-CT scan.

During you and your child's first visit, the doctor will ask you to complete a **medical history** on your child. If this is your child's regular doctor, the doctor may already have some of this information. Your responsibility is to provide the doctor with information that is *complete, accurate, truthful, and up-to-date*. This information is the foundation on which the doctor will begin to make a diagnosis.

You should be prepared to answer the following types of questions:

Your child's and family's medical history. Do allergies or asthma run in your family? Has your child suffered recurrent respiratory infections? Does the child have any known allergic disorders? For example, does your child have hayfever, sinus infections, skin problems (atopic dermatitis), or reactions to foods, drugs, etc.? Has the child had recurrent nosebleeds or loss of smell or taste?

Symptoms. Does your child experience coughing, wheezing, shortness of breath, chest tightness, and coughing up phlegm? Are the symptoms associated with seasons or do they occur year-round? How often do symptoms occur? How severe are they? Do symptoms occur more frequently at night?

Progress of the disease. When did your child's symptoms begin? Has the disease gotten better or worse over time? Has the child ever been evaluated by a doctor for asthma? If so, what was the result? If your child has been previously diagnosed with asthma, how are you currently managing his or her condition? What medications is he or she currently taking?

Severity of the disease. How many times in the past year has your child visited the emergency room, urgent care center, or been hospitalized for asthma-related symptoms? Has your child ever had a life-threatening asthma episode? How many days of school has your child missed this year due to asthma symptoms? Do symptoms limit his or her physical activities? How often does your child have nighttime asthma? How has the condition affected your child's growth, behavior, lifestyle, and school achievement?

Factors that may aggravate the condition. What factors trigger or make the asthma symptoms worse:

- Viral respiratory infections?

- Environmental allergens (pollen, mold, dust mites, cockroaches, and animal dander, saliva, or urine)?

- Changes in environment (moving to a new home, going on vacation, and/or changes in school environment)?

- Exposure to irritants (tobacco smoke, strong odors, air pollutants, chemicals, vapors, gases, and aerosols)?

- Strong emotions (fear, anxiety, anger, crying, laughing)?

- Drugs (aspirin or other non-steroidal anti-inflammatory drugs (NSAIDs), or others)?

- Food additives and preservatives (monosodium glutamate (MSG), sulfites, yellow dye No. 5)?

- Changes in the weather or cold air?

- Exercise?

- Others?

Your child's living environment. Are there animals in your home? Do you have carpets in the home? Is your child exposed to second-hand smoke or does the child himself smoke? Does your home have an air conditioner, central heat, and/or a humidifier?

The doctor will perform a **physical exam** on your child to assess his or her overall health. In addition, the doctor will likely examine the skin for signs of *hives* or *eczema*, the ears for signs of *inflammation*, the eyes for *dark circles* (allergic shiners), the chest (lungs, heart, diaphragm) for symptoms of *wheezing/obstructed airflow* or physical clues like *hunched shoulders* and *exaggerated development of the chest* (pigeon chest), and the nose and throat for *inflammation, sinusitis, nasal polyps* (noncancerous growths in the nose), or *structural abnormalities*.

Next, your doctor will likely perform breathing tests to see how well your child's lungs are functioning. This can be done with a simple hand-held device called a peak flow meter or a more complicated machine called a spirometer. The child blows out (exhales) as much air as he or she can in one second (one-second vital capacity test). A child whose airways are narrowed due to asthma will be able to blow out less air than a child without asthma. (The peak flow meter is a useful home monitoring tool. See "How Can a Peak Flow Meter Help Me Manage My Child's Asthma?" on page 32.)

Your doctor may use a more sophisticated lung-function measuring device like a spirometer, which is a closed tube connected to a machine. It measures how much air the lungs can hold (lung volume) as well as how much air your child can exhale. The results are recorded on graph paper, which the doctor can then analyze.

The doctor may also give your child a **bronchospasm evaluation,** in which the child inhales a bronchodilator drug that acts to open up the airways, and then exhales into a peak flow meter or spirometer. If your child's lung function improves significantly, chances are good the child has asthma.

During follow-up visits, your doctor will use the peak flow meter or the spirometer to evaluate your child's condition and to see how well his or her treatment plan is working.

After the doctor has performed these and other lung-function tests, he or she may want to take an **x-ray** of your child's chest. Although a chest x-ray isn't vital to diagnosing asthma, it can rule out cystic fibrosis, a rare lung condition that causes the lungs to become clogged with thick mucus and results in recurrent infections and pneumonia.

A chest x-ray can also reveal a relatively common cause of childhood wheezing: a foreign object or food that becomes stuck in the windpipe. Children, especially toddlers, have a habit of placing everything they come in contact with into their mouths. Foreign objects or food can be inhaled into the lungs and become lodged in the trachea or bronchial tubes, where they can cause wheezing that mimics asthma. Regular chest x-rays can't always reveal foreign objects. If the x-ray is negative, the doctor may have to use a special instrument called a bronchoscope to look directly into the bronchial tubes to locate and remove the object.

A chest x-ray may also be a good idea if your child has a respiratory infection. The chest x-ray can help the doctor determine the extent and severity of the infection.

In addition, your child's doctor will likely want to take a **sinus x-ray** to determine whether or not your child has sinus disease. A plain x-ray may be helpful or a more sensitive CAT scan may be needed, especially if the small sinuses around the eyes are involved.

Your doctor may also want to perform a variety of **laboratory tests** on your child. These may include a *sputum* or *nasal smear*. The doctor will examine mucus from the nose or chest under a microscope to see if there are larger-than-normal levels of eosinophils, white blood cells that indicate asthma or an ongoing allergic reaction.

Blood tests can also help diagnose asthma. The doctor will look for sufficient numbers of white blood cells and check the numbers of eosinophils, special white blood cells. If your child has asthma, he or she may have a lower number of the white blood cells that fight infection and a higher number of eosinophils. The doctor may also want to test the blood for oxygen blood levels or the amount of immunoglobulin E (IgE), proteins which are associated with asthma.

If your doctor suspects that your child's symptoms are related to allergies, he or she may refer your child to an allergist for **allergy skin testing**. These tests can identify specific allergens so they can be avoided. The doctor uses a very concentrated liquid extract of a suspected allergen such as house dust. He or she places a drop of the allergen extract on the child's skin and then scratches or pricks the skin. This is not a painful experience and the test does not draw blood. If the child is allergic to the substance, a red, itchy welt will develop around the test site. The size of the welt reflects your child's sensitivity to the substance. The welt will then go away in a short period of time. (When scratch or prick tests are normal and the doctor still suspects the child is allergic, he or she may use an intradermal test, in which a small amount of the allergen is injected under the skin.)

Usually, the doctor will test for common allergens such as molds, dust mites, animal dander, and grass and tree pollens. However, nearly any substance can be tested. Be sure to request tests for substances you suspect to be allergens for your child. Testing only takes a short time and results are usually available within 20 to 30 minutes. These tests help the doctor advise parents about what triggers to avoid and what household items may help. Sometimes, avoidance of certain allergens may be impossible, in which case your doctor may suggest immunotherapy.

Your child may also be reactive to certain foods, food additives or preservatives. Unfortunately, because children usually eat a varied diet and dishes are often combinations of several foods, sensitivities to particular foods aren't always easily identified. If the allergist suspects your child reacts to specific foods, he or she may simply suggest eliminating those foods from the diet and watching the results.

How Severe Is My Child's Asthma?

Experts classify asthma by severity: Mild (episodic), Moderate (chronic), and Severe (chronic). This allows them to categorize all of the information about your child's condition and select the right treatment. Because asthma varies widely among different children, the characteristics that classify a child's asthma as mild, moderate, or severe may overlap and your child may, over time, switch into different classifications.

The asthma classification chart on the next page was adapted from the National Institutes of Health's National Asthma Education Program.

Asthma Classification Chart

Characteristic	Mild	Moderate	Severe
Frequency of attacks	Coughing, wheezing no more than 1-2 times/wk.	Coughing, wheezing more than 2 times/wk. Urgent hospital or doctor's office care less than 3 times/yr.	Daily wheezing. Frequent, severe attacks. Urgent hospital or doctor's care more than 3 times/yr.
Frequency of symptoms	Few symptoms between attacks.	Cough, wheezing between attacks.	Continuous cough, wheezing.
Exercise tolerance	Good. May not tolerate vigorous exercise.	Diminished tolerance.	Poor tolerance. Limited activity.
Frequency of nighttime asthma	No more than 1-2 times/mo.	1-3 times/wk.	Almost nightly symptoms.
School/work attendance	Good.	Attendance may be affected.	Poor attendance.
Peak flow meter reading	Greater than 80% of predicted value; varies less than 20%.	60-80% of predicted value; varies 20-30%.	Less than 60% of predicted value; varies greater than 30%.

Source: Adapted from the National Institutes of Health National Asthma Education Program.

Professional Help: an Essential Part of Managing Your Child's Asthma

Childhood asthma is not something you can self-treat without a health care professional's help. Too often, parents don't realize their child's coughing, wheezing, recurrent respiratory infections, and other symptoms are caused by asthma, a serious condition that requires regular medical care. In fact, the increase in childhood asthma deaths in recent years has been blamed, in part, on caregivers not taking the disease seriously enough and not getting the right treatment.

No matter how much you learn about your child's asthma, it won't be enough. Your health care team will know more. They have the advantage of years of training and daily practical experience. They have access to the latest medical literature, the newest medicines, and the most up-to-date technology for treating your child's condition.

Much of the day-to-day responsibility for managing your child's asthma will fall on you. However, you'll need providers who can guide you and monitor your child's treatment. You'll need a doctor with whom you can communicate openly to develop a treatment plan together that's right for your child. This is where teamwork among you, your child, the doctor, and other members of your health care team can make an important difference in asthma control.

How Can I Find the Right Doctor for My Child?

Choosing a doctor is never easy, but choosing a pediatrician for a child who has asthma is even more difficult. You need a doctor who is a good children's doctor and one who is also knowledgeable about children's asthma.

If you are a member of a managed care organization, you may feel your freedom to select or choose a doctor is limited. However, this is not necessarily true. Your freedom begins when you select your health care coverage. If you have a choice among different plans, research the plan and the doctors associated with the plan *before* you enroll. Even if you don't have a choice of plans, you are still able to choose a doctor within your plan. Talk with possible providers about your child's condition and their approach. Also, learn what other kinds of providers they may refer you to, if special care is needed in managing your child's condition.

You may already have a pediatrician you and your child know and trust. If so, start with him or her. Your doctor may refer your child to an allergy or lung specialist if needed.

If you don't have a pediatrician who can treat your child's asthma, here are some tips in choosing the right one:

Make a list of pediatricians. Ask everyone you know about their children's doctors—friends, relatives, coworkers. Find out why they like the doctor. If your town has a community hospital or a large teaching hospital, call and ask for names of pediatricians. You can also ask your local chapter of the American Lung Association for names of doctors who treat children's asthma.

Make an appointment. Some doctors will take a few moments for a brief phone interview. Others will want you to come in.

Ask questions. At your initial visit, ask questions that will help you assess whether or not this doctor is qualified to treat your child's asthma:

- What training and experience have you had in treating childhood asthma?

- What are your beliefs about asthma treatment? (Doctors have different ideas about how asthma should be treated and managed.)

- Will you refer patients to allergists for skin testing and immunotherapy?

- What do you think the role of the parents should be in a child's asthma management?

- How do you feel about the use of home peak flow meters and other self-management strategies?

- Are you available for consultation by phone? Do you charge for phone consultation?

- Are you available for emergencies?

- Where do you have hospital privileges?

Trust your "gut" feeling. It won't take long during your initial visit for you to get a feel for the fit between your doctor's personality and personal style and you and your child's. Did this doctor seem truly interested and concerned about your child's welfare? Was the doctor empathetic? Did the doctor allow you to ask questions and did he or she provide understandable answers? Did the doctor speak in plain language or use "medic speak"? Did you have enough time, or did the doctor make you feel rushed? Do you like this doctor?

Ask your child's opinion. If your child is old enough, include him or her in the decision about who will treat his or her condition.

Will My Child Need to See Specialists?

The pediatrician is your child's primary care doctor. He or she should supervise the treatment of your child's asthma. This is the doctor who should coordinate with specialists and other health care providers to make sure your child is getting the care he or she needs.

The pediatrician may be able to treat your child's condition successfully. After all, asthma is a common disease, and many doctors who aren't asthma specialists are able to do a good job of diagnosing or managing it. However, he or she may want your child to see an asthma specialist. Or you may feel your child needs more help than the pediatrician is able to provide. Asthma specialists don't take the place of your child's pediatrician. The pediatrician still oversees your child's therapy. Asthma specialists, however, can help refine your child's treatment and make sure he or she is getting exactly the right therapy.

These are some of the other professionals who might be on your child's asthma health care team:

Allergist. If the doctor believes your child's asthma is related to allergies, he or she might refer your child to an allergist. An allergist is a medical doctor with specialized training in allergy and immunology and asthma management. An allergist can conduct allergy testing to pinpoint exactly what your child is allergic to and provide practical advice in avoiding allergens. The allergist can also give your child allergy shots (immunotherapy) that can help reduce his or her sensitivity to those allergens that can't be avoided.

Pulmonologist. Also called a pulmonary specialist, a pulmonologist is a medical doctor with specialized training in and knowledge about respiratory disorders. Because these doctors are lung specialists, chances are good that they are knowledgeable about the latest medicines, tests, technology, and treatments for your child's asthma.

Working With My Child's Health Care Team

Most of us come out of the "Yes, Doctor" school of communication. Confronted with a person in a white coat, we seem to lose our ability to speak up, to ask questions, to get our concerns addressed. When a health care professional says something we don't understand, instead of asking for clarification, we simply say "Yes, Doctor."

As a parent of a child with asthma, you're going to have to teach yourself how to communicate with your child's health care team. Your child depends on you. You are his or her advocate with the health care system. You are the major source of information about your child's condition, and your child's doctor, nurse, pharmacist, and other health care providers must rely on you for accurate, up-to-date information. To help your child manage his or her asthma, you're going to have to establish a partnership with this team and your child, one that has honest and open communication.

Here are a few tips on how to do that:

Talk about your fears and your concerns up front. Common sense says and research has confirmed that parents are able to focus fully on the treatment only after they've addressed their major concerns with a health care professional. What are your biggest fears? What is the worst thing you can imagine happening? What is the best possible outcome for your child? Are you concerned about money or your ability to manage the treatment regimen? Do you have fears about your child's emotional reactions to his or her condition?

Be clear about your goals and expectations. Doctors aren't miracle workers, and medicine isn't magic. Often parents are dissatisfied with the provider or the treatment because their goals and expectations are unrealistic considering the severity of the child's illness. Talk with the provider about what you expect from the treatment. What exactly does "controlling" your child's asthma mean? Will your child be symptom-free with treatment, or is he or she likely to experience frequent symptoms and episodes?

Establish your respective roles. Another source of potential conflict between you and the members of your health care team are your expectations about your roles. Be clear about what each of your jobs will be in managing your child's asthma. The easiest way to do this is to talk honestly about it. Ask them: "What is my role in managing my child's asthma? What is it you expect me and my child to do?" Also talk about what the other team members' roles are.

Be honest. Your providers can't do the best job for your child if they don't have accurate and up-to-date information. Talk with them honestly about your child's condition, your family environment, and lifestyle factors that may affect your child's asthma. For example, if you smoke or your child smokes, tell them. This information can affect your child's asthma treatment.

Today, many teenagers and even younger children are experimenting with illegal drugs. Many of these drugs can have an adverse impact on a child's asthma. For example, smoking marijuana or crack can irritate the bronchial tubes and bring on asthma attacks. Cocaine or uppers can have dangerous interactions with certain asthma drugs. If you think your child might be using drugs of any kind, tell your doctor. (Information you give your doctor is confidential.) He or she can offer resources that can help.

Let your child's health care team know if you or your child are having difficulty sticking with any part of your child's treatment program. It's quite common for young teenagers to go through a rebellious period where they refuse or "forget" to take their medication or monitor their condition. Providers may be able to help with strategies that can make working with your child's treatment plan easier and more effective.

Ask all members of your health care team to speak in plain language. Many health care professionals are quite able to explain complex medical topics in understandable language. Others are not so skilled. If your provider uses "medic speak" that you or your child don't understand, ask him or her to explain it in simpler terms or draw you a picture. Never go away not understanding what your provider is saying.

Get your questions answered. You have the right to ask questions and get answers you can understand. If you don't ask questions, your provider might assume you already know. Ask and keep asking until you understand. Remember, the only question that is "dumb" is the one that goes unasked and unanswered. Your health care team can provide pamphlets with information about asthma that you can take home. Some provide video cassettes for home loan as well. Guidelines for therapy should be written out for the patient.

Give information. Let your child's health care team know about the frequency and severity of your child's symptoms. Tell them what makes symptoms worse or better. Give them feedback about how the treatment is working, including any side effects.

Questions You Should Ask Your Child's Doctor

Testing. What does each of these tests do? How are they performed? How much do they cost? Are all of them necessary?

Diagnosis. What does this diagnosis mean? What do you mean by mild, moderate, or severe asthma?

Severity of condition. How will my child's condition affect his or her lifestyle, including school attendance and physical activity?

Warning signs. What are the warning signs I should look out for, and what should I do if I see them?

Medications. What is the name of this drug (generic and brand name)? What is it for? How should my child take this drug and how often? What are the risks? What are the possible side effects? Should I report all side effects to you? What precautions are necessary while taking this drug, and are there any special instructions about food or possible drug interactions? What should we do if my child misses a dose?

Follow-up appointments. How often does my child need to see you?

How Can I Get the Most from Doctor Visits?

There's nothing worse than taking your child to the doctor's office, being kept waiting, and then leaving feeling like you didn't get what you wanted from the visit. A little pre-visit preparation can make your child's visits to the doctor more productive.

Prepare an agenda. You'll get more from the visit if you know what you want from it ahead of time. Take some time to think about what it is you want to accomplish at the next visit. Maybe you want the doctor to reevaluate your child's medication or demonstrate how to use a peak flow meter. Perhaps you need information about support groups or asthma camps. Or maybe you need help in coping with your child's emotional reactions to his or her condition.

Take a notebook. Jot down your concerns, your questions, and your goals for your doctor's appointment in a notebook and bring it with you. That way you won't leave without getting what you and your child need.

Don't waste time. Neither your time nor the doctor's is unlimited. Your life is busy, and the doctor probably has hundreds of people depending on him or her. Keep your conversation during office visits relevant to your child's condition. Don't waste time with chitchat. Be specific, concise, and direct in your comments.

Write down the doctor's instructions. Then read them back to make sure you have them right. Or take along a tape recorder and tape the session.

Bring along your partner, a relative, or a friend as a second set of ears. It's helpful to be able to talk about your child's treatment and the results of the latest visit, especially with your partner. However, if your partner isn't available, take along a trusted friend or relative. They can help you keep track of the issues you want to discuss and the doctor's instructions. This second pair of ears is particularly helpful during an emergency situation such as a serious asthma episode.

Developing a Treatment Plan with the Health Care Team

One of the most important responsibilities you have as a parent of a child with asthma is to work closely with providers and jointly develop a written treatment plan (also called a management plan) for controlling your child's asthma. No one's asthma is the same, and no two children will have the same treatment plan. Your child's treatment must be individualized to fit him or her. It must be **simple**, so that you and your family can carry out the instructions. Yet it must be **detailed**, so that you know exactly what to do to prevent asthma episodes and what to do when asthma symptoms do occur.

Your doctor should **write down** your treatment plan so that you can refer to it when you need it. He or she should **review it** with you to ensure you understand it and are able to comply with the instructions. And you and the doctor should periodically (every six to twelve months) go over the treatment plan and make changes as needed.

If you don't yet have a written treatment plan for your child, don't hesitate to ask your doctor about one. Having a treatment plan will help you feel more confident and less fearful about your child's condition. It will help you know what to do to help your child, no matter how mild or how serious the asthma symptoms might be. It can also help you to reduce and/or eliminate your child's symptoms, and use less medicine to keep symptoms in check or to recover from an asthma episode.

Be sure to share your child's treatment plan with school officials, child care providers, or anyone else who might provide care for your child. Include your child in these meetings if he or she is old enough.

Your child's treatment plan may vary, but it should contain these elements:

Information about medicines. The plan should include what the medication is (generic and brand name), what it does, how much to take, how often to take it, and possible side effects and when to report them to the doctor. It should provide guidelines about changing a dose or adding medications, if appropriate, and what to do if your child misses a dose.

Early warning signs to watch for. Early warning signs vary among children, but, by observing carefully, you'll soon learn the signs that precede an episode for your child. By recognizing these signs early, you'll be able to start treatment early and possibly prevent an asthma episode.

Peak flow meter monitoring guidelines. If you and your child are monitoring his or her condition with a peak flow meter, the treatment plan should list peak expiratory flow rate (PEFR) values that indicate airflow obstruction.

When to begin treatment and specifically what treatment to use. Your child's treatment plan shouldn't leave you wondering what to do. It should specifically tell you what medicines to use and what actions to take.

Steps to manage an asthma episode. Nothing is quite as frightening as a full-blown asthma flare. Your management plan should tell you, step by step, how to respond.

Guidelines for seeking emergency help. Parents often wait too long before seeking emergency help for their child with asthma. Your plan should tell you what signs to watch for so you can seek emergency help.

Signs that your child's treatment plan needs to be reevaluated. Treatment plans aren't static and neither is your child's asthma. Your plan should include signs that indicate your child may need a change in treatment.

Emergency names, numbers and addresses. Don't wait until there is an emergency to make information about the doctor, hospital, ambulance, friend or relative to call, and emergency transportation part of your child's treatment plan. A note to the teacher or coach is often needed so that the child may use his or her inhaler before exercise.

You can get an idea of what a treatment plan might look like by reviewing this sample plan adapted from the National Asthma Education Program.

Sample Treatment Plan

Mild Episode

Symptoms: Mild wheezing, coughing, chest tightness, shortness of breath, with activity.

Peak flow: 70-90% of personal best.

Actions to take: Use inhaled bronchodilator. If symptoms improve, continue regularly for 24-48 hours. If no improvement, see action under Moderate Episode.

Moderate Episode

Symptoms: Wheezing, coughing, shortness of breath, at rest.

Peak flow: 50-70% of personal best.

Actions to take: Use inhaled bronchodilator every 20 minutes for 1 hour. If there is improvement, continue every 3-4 hours for 24-48 hours. If no improvement in 2-6 hours, begin or increase prednisone. Contact doctor.

Severe Episode

Symptoms: Severe shortness of breath, wheezing, coughing, chest tightness at rest. Difficulty walking or talking. Possible retraction of neck or chest muscles.

Peak flow: Less than 50% of personal best. Little response to bronchodilator.

Actions to take: Use 4-6 puffs of inhaled bronchodilator every 10 minutes, up to 3 times. Begin or increase prednisone. Call doctor. If no improvement in 20-30 minutes, seek emergency help.

Doctor: _____ Telephone: _____

Address: _____

Hospital: _____ Telephone: _____

Address: _____

Ambulance: _____ Telephone: _____

Address: _____

Friend/relative: _____ Telephone: _____

Address: _____

Taxi: _____ Telephone: _____

Address: _____

How Can a Peak Flow Meter Help Me Manage My Child's Asthma?

A peak flow meter is an inexpensive hand-held device that even young children (5 years and older) can use to monitor the flow of air through the lungs. Previously, peak flow meters were only used in lung specialists' offices. More recently, however, they've become a valuable self-management tool for use at home. Regular use of a peak flow meter can help you and your child:

Provide an objective measurement of how the lungs are functioning. It's difficult for the child, the parent, or even the doctor to tell how a child's lungs are doing without measuring the air flow out of the lungs.

Monitor changes in lung function. Asthma doesn't behave the same way 24 hours a day. Often, asthma is better during the day and worse at night. Children can get into trouble with their asthma when a doctor isn't around. By the time they see the doctor in the office the following day, the asthma is likely improved.

Avoid unnecessary doctor's office or hospital visits. Peak flow meter readings allow you to call the doctor with specific, objective information and get advice on how to respond. Often, the doctor can help get the child out of trouble with a simple phone call, without an office or emergency room visit.

Measure the stability of the child's condition. When the child's peak flow meter readings don't vary widely, it's a clue that the child's condition is currently stable and isn't getting worse or better.

Anticipate asthma attacks. A peak flow meter reading that drops by 20 percent or more is an indication that the child stands a good chance of getting into trouble with his or her asthma within the next 24 hours. The readings allow you to refer to your treatment plan or to consult your doctor and respond quickly before the symptoms get worse.

Evaluate how medications are working. Peak flow meter readings can help the doctor adjust the drugs and the doses to help your child maintain normal lung function. Only when the child is having less than one asthma episode a week should bronchodilators be used solely as rescue therapy. Since we now know that thickening of the lung basement membranes begins with even mild asthma, anti-inflammatory medicines should always be available.

Identify asthma "triggers." Regularly using the peak flow meter can help you and your child determine what triggers, or brings on, your child's symptoms. This enables you to help your child avoid his or her personal asthma triggers.

Keep yourself and your child motivated. Sometimes following your child's treatment plan day after day can be difficult. Keeping track of peak flow meter readings and watching the readings improve as you and your child get his or her asthma under control can serve as a motivational tool. With young children, you can make a game of taking and recording peak flow meter readings and use incentives like stars, smile faces, or other symbols in their personal peak flow meter log.

According to the Asthma and Allergy Foundation of America, you should have your child keep and use a home peak flow meter if any of the following situations occur:

• Your child experiences severe asthma attacks with little warning.

• Your child's condition requires use of the medications cromolyn and/or (low-dose) inhaled corticosteroids, and there are special circumstances such as traveling long distances for medical attention.

• Your child requires high-dose inhaled corticosteroids or daily oral corticosteroids.

• Your child has big swings (greater than 20 percent) in his or her peak flow meter readings at the doctor's office.

• Your child's asthma history isn't a reliable guide for treatment. Many patients are unaware of their disease, and many lungs are silent when listened to with a stethoscope. So, new asthma guidelines suggest that both peak flow meters and spirometry should be part of every asthmatic child's routine exam, as soon as they are old enough for the tests.

How to Use a Peak Flow Meter

It's easy to learn to use a peak flow meter.

1. Set the peak flow meter marker to zero.

2. Have your child stand up straight.

3. Tell the child to take a deep breath.

4. Have the child place the meter in his or her mouth, closing lips around the mouthpiece (make sure the child's tongue doesn't block the mouthpiece).

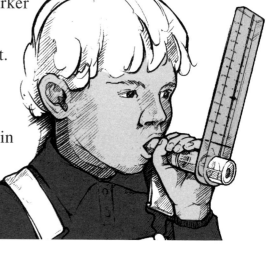

5. Have the child breathe out quickly and forcefully through the mouth into the flow meter.

6. Record the reading.

7. Reset the peak flow meter marker back to zero and have the child repeat two more times. If your child is doing it right, there should be little change in his or her readings.

8. Record the highest reading on your child's peak flow diary chart. Include the date, time, peak flow meter reading, and any other notes you think might be important (such as exposure to triggers).

9. Clean the mouthpiece daily. Wash your hands, then remove and disassemble, or take apart, the washable parts of the meter, and wash in warm water (don't use bleach, vinegar, or very hot water). Shake off excess moisture and allow to air dry. When the equipment is completely dry, store in a clean, sealed plastic bag.

For Best Results When Using the Peak Flow Meter:

- Ask your doctor or nurse to instruct you and your child in the correct use of a peak flow meter. Have your child practice using the device in the doctor's office to ensure he or she is using it correctly. Ask the doctor to recheck correct usage periodically.

- Have your doctor or nurse help you to determine your child's personal best or baseline peak flow meter reading. This will be the figure against which you'll judge all other peak flow meter readings.

  ➤ Measure and record your child's peak expiratory flow rate twice a day, morning and evening, for two to three weeks. Record the highest number from each session.

  ➤ Take the reading before and after the child takes inhaled medications.

  ➤ Share the readings with the doctor, who will help you determine your child's personal best figure. This is usually an evening reading taken after the child has taken the maximum dose of medication prescribed.

  ➤ Have your child's personal best peak flow meter readings reevaluated at least annually by the doctor.

- Record measurements daily (or as instructed by the doctor), morning and evening, in your child's peak flow meter log.

- Always have your child perform three peak flow meter exhalations and record the highest.

- If your child's asthma is stable and your doctor recommends taking only sporadic readings, take them both on the same day, morning and evening.

- Measure changes in your child's peak flow meter readings against his or her personal best reading. Then follow the instructions outlined in your child's treatment plan.

- As the child gets older, make taking his or her peak expiratory flow readings part of the daily chores. Reward the child just as you would for other good behavior.

- Use the "traffic light" system to interpret results (see page 37).

Peak Flow Meter Readings

Ask your doctor to provide you with a chart or log to record your child's peak flow meter readings, or use the one provided here.

Date																
Time	AM		PM	AM		PM	AM		PM	AM		PM	AM		PM	AM		PM
600																
575																
550																
525																
500																
475																
450																
425																
400																
375																
350																
325																
300																
275																
250																
225																
200																
175																
150																
125																
100																
75																
50																
25																
0																

What Do Peak Flow Meter Readings Mean?

It's easy to interpret your child's peak flow meter readings with the **traffic light** system doctors have devised. Readings are divided into **green** ("All Clear"), **yellow** ("Caution"), and **red** ("Stop: Medical Emergency"). A normal peak flow rate can vary as much as 20 percent. Your child's peak flow meter readings will be measured against his or her personal best reading. *Declines of more than 20 percent of this figure indicate a need for more medication.*

Your doctor may suggest other zones to follow, especially if your child's asthma worsens rapidly. For example, your doctor may have your child's yellow zone start at 90 percent of his or her personal best.

Green, or 80 to 100 percent of personal best. This is an "all clear" signal. Your child has no asthma symptoms, and you can plan on following your child's routine management plan. If your child is taking medications regularly and has consistently "green" readings, ask your doctor to reevaluate his or her treatment plan. It may be that your child will be able to reduce medication (never reduce medications without the doctor's instructions or approval).

Yellow, or 50 to 80 percent of personal best. This is a "caution" signal. It means that your child's airways are narrowing and may need extra treatment. Follow the instructions for this zone in your child's treatment plan. If the readings and/or symptoms don't improve with medication, call the doctor.

A decrease in peak flow of 20 to 30 percent of your child's personal best may mean the start of an asthma episode. Follow your treatment plan instructions for treating an asthma episode.

Readings in the caution zone may also indicate your child's asthma is not well controlled. Talk with the doctor about reevaluating your child's maintenance medication.

Red, or below 50 percent of personal best. *Stop! This is a medical emergency.* Give your child a bronchodilator medication immediately. Contact the doctor immediately if the peak expiratory flow rate measurements don't quickly return and stay in the yellow or green zones.

Peak Flow Meter Traffic System

If your child uses a peak flow meter, a treatment plan might look like this one adapted from the National Asthma Education Program:

GREEN ZONE: All Clear

Peak flow is _____ (80 to 100 percent of your child's personal best). No symptoms are present; your child can do his or her usual activities and sleep without symptoms.

Medications: Have your child take these medications:

Medication_____ Dosage_____ When_____

Medication_____ Dosage_____ When_____

Control triggers: Follow the treatment plan to avoid things that bring on your child's asthma.

Exercise: Take _____ (medication) before exercise.

YELLOW ZONE: Caution

Peak flow is _____ (50 to 80 percent of your child's personal best). Symptoms may be mild or moderate. Your child may cough, wheeze, feel short of breath, or feel like his or her chest is tight. Symptoms may keep the child from regular activities or sleep.

Medication: Take this medicine first.

Medication_____ Dosage_____ When_____

If your child feels better in 20 to 60 minutes and peak flow is over _____, take the medicine listed below.

Medication_____ Dosage_____ When_____

Keep having the child take his or her green zone medications.

If your child DOES NOT feel better in 20 to 60 minutes or peak flow is under _____, **follow red zone plan.**

(If your child keeps going into the yellow zone, talk with your doctor. Your child's green zone medications may need to be changed).

Peak Flow Meter Traffic System

RED ZONE: Stop! Medical Emergency!

This is a medical emergency! Get help! Your child's asthma symptoms are serious. The peak flow meter reading is _____ (below 50 percent of personal best). Your child may be coughing, very short of breath, and/or the skin between the ribs and neck may be pulled tight. Your child may have trouble walking or talking. The child may not wheeze because he or she cannot move air out of the airways.

Medication: Take this medication first.

Medication_____ Dosage_____ When_____

Call the doctor: Ask the doctor what you should do next. Tell him or her this is an emergency.

Get emergency medical help: Get to a doctor or hospital right away if any of these things are happening:

- Your child's lips or fingernails are blue.

- Your child is struggling to breathe.

- Your child does not feel any better 20 to 30 minutes after taking the extra medicine and his or her peak flow meter reading is still under _____ (50 percent of personal best).

- Your child has taken the extra medication and six hours later still needs inhaled beta$_2$-agonist medicine every one to three hours and his or her peak flow is under _____ (70 percent of personal best).

Getting the Most from Asthma Medications

One of the biggest problems with children, especially adolescents, is getting them to take their medication on time and in the right dosage. Obviously, the responsibility will fall on you when your child is young. As your child gets older, he or she will need to assume more responsibility for taking the asthma medications as prescribed.

A chronic disease like asthma can be tough on children. It can make them feel different from other children. They may feel like all they do is take medications. It will be one of your biggest jobs to help your child learn about his or her condition and how to manage it, and to teach him or her the importance of following the treatment plan, including taking medications.

Doctors prescribe asthma medications to prevent episodes from occurring, to keep early symptoms from progressing into a full-blown flare, and to treat asthma episodes when they occur. A few years ago, treatment for asthma focused primarily on preventing the airway muscles from tightening (bronchospasm). While it's still important to control bronchospasms, doctors have discovered it's also important to control and/or prevent the underlying inflammation of the airways that leads to asthma symptoms. Your child's doctor may prescribe anti-inflammatory drugs like low-dose inhaled corticosteroids, cromolyn, or, if your child's asthma is very severe, oral corticosteroids.

Since your child's asthma is unique to him or her, the drugs the doctor prescribes should be tailored to your child's individualized needs. What works for your child's friend may not work for your child. It may take some trial and error before you and your doctor find exactly the right combination of drugs. And those drugs may have to be changed as newer, more effective medications become available, and as your child's condition changes.

Asthma medications come in liquids, powders, pills, injections, and inhaled vapors. Some children take the same drugs in different ways. For example, a very young child may take his or her asthma medication through a compressor-driven device called a nebulizer. An older child may take the same medication with a hand-held metered dose inhaler. Some children must take regular daily doses of asthma medications to control their condition. Others may take medications only when early warning signs appear, or before they're exposed to one of their known asthma triggers such as animal dander or exercise. Still other children take regular doses of asthma medications with higher doses or additional drugs when exposed to triggers or when symptoms appear.

Here are some tips for helping your child get the most from his or her asthma medications and some ideas to help you as a parent see that your child takes his medication on time and in the right dose.

Link taking medications to consequences. Even small children learn quickly about the consequences of their actions. Touch a hot stove, burn your hand. Eat too much candy, get a stomach ache. Likewise, children can be taught that there are positive consequences for taking medications (feeling good, without symptoms) and negative consequences (feeling bad, coughing, wheezing, chest tightness, and possibly hospitalization) for not taking them. Help your child see that taking his or her medications and complying with other aspects of the management program mean the freedom to feel good and do things other children do.

Teach your child about the reality of asthma. You don't want to scare your child, but you also do want your child to understand that asthma is a serious disease that can be controlled with proper management. Impress on your child that taking medications is an important step in managing this health problem.

Use positive rewards. Set up a system of positive rewards that reinforces your child's taking his or her medication. Perhaps it's a video the child's been wanting to see, or a special item of clothing, or an activity the child enjoys. After a period (a week or a month) of taking the medications on time and in the right amount, reward the child.

Keep it simple. Help the child remember his or her medications by creating a simple system such as color-coding medication bottles, setting out medications with breakfast, or attaching notes.

Keep a positive attitude. Frustration and depression at times are part of any chronic disease. Try to avoid the negative aspects, and take a positive approach to your child's asthma. In most cases, your child's attitude about the disease will reflect your own. Learning to control his or her asthma can help your child gain confidence and learn self-discipline and responsibility.

Make age-appropriate changes. Children can take the same asthma medications as adults, with certain modifications. For example, for infants or very young children, you'll probably have to administer medications using a nebulizer with a face mask. As children get older and are able to use hand-held inhalers, they can use spacers—medicine holding chambers that make using inhalers easier. Children who have difficulty taking oral medications can be given syrups or other forms such as Theo-Dur Sprinkles. Or you can mix the medication with a spoonful of applesauce. Talk with your doctor about other solutions if you have trouble getting your child to take medication.

Have your child take the medication exactly as the doctor prescribes. Your child's treatment plan should outline when to take the medication, how to take it, and what to do if he or she misses a dose.

Don't give your child more medication than the doctor recommends. Increasing your child's medication without your doctor's approval can be dangerous. The wrong dose can cause dangerous side effects.

Don't allow your child to skip medication because he or she is feeling well. Most asthma drugs are best taken preventively and regularly. Chronic airway inflammation, which is present even in mild asthma, makes your child vulnerable to an asthma flare. Using medications preventively can decrease the irritation and give your child some protection against an asthma episode. The child should understand that the anti-inflammatory medicine, no matter what kind, is crucial to healing of the lungs. The bronchodilator is no substitute for this.

Give your child medications promptly when early symptoms occur. Make sure your child takes his or her medications within five minutes after experiencing the first symptom.

Help your child take responsibility for knowing the names of all his or her medications and taking them properly.

Be sure your child keeps an inhaler on hand at all times. You never know when your child will need to "rescue" his or her airways from the beginnings of an episode.

Be sure your doctor and pharmacist know all the drugs your child is taking. Even over-the-counter drugs can cause problems.

Help your child avoid taking illegal drugs. Street drugs can play havoc with your child's asthma treatment. Marijuana and crack both irritate the airways. Downers and other types of depressants can inhibit your child's breathing. Any mind-altering drug can make it difficult for your child to take his or her medication at the right time and in the correct dose. Talk frankly with your child about so-called recreational drugs.

Give your child the facts about smoking. Many children, especially young adolescents, are tempted to smoke cigarettes. Smoke from tobacco products is particularly dangerous to an asthmatic.

Be alert for side effects and report them promptly to your doctor. Know the possible side effects of each drug. If your child is having side effects, call the doctor. If you can't reach your doctor or pharmacist, reduce your child's next dose by one-half or skip the dose. Do not allow your child to stop taking his or her medication entirely without talking with the doctor.

Have your child take oral medications according to directions to reduce side effects. Some drugs are best taken before meals, some with meals. Other drugs are unaffected by food.

When taking inhaled corticosteroids, be sure your child rinses his or her mouth and throat by swallowing water after taking. This simple step can help reduce your child's chances of getting a yeast infection in the mouth (thrush).

Have patience. Don't expect medications to make your child feel better instantly. Some of them take weeks to take effect. Know what to expect, and report to the doctor if your child's treatment isn't working.

Store medications properly. Your doctor or pharmacist can tell you if any of your child's medications have special storage instructions. In most cases, drugs should be stored in a cool, dark, dry place. Do not store them in the bathroom (it's not cool or dry there), near the stove or oven, in the car, or anywhere young children might find them.

How Can a Metered Dose Inhaler Help My Child?

A metered dose inhaler (MDI) is a pressurized canister, like a tiny spray can, of medication that is inserted into a holder with a mouthpiece. It delivers a measured (metered) dose of medication that comes out as a fine mist or spray. Many asthma medications are now administered by MDI. There are fewer side effects when the drug is delivered right to the lungs rather than to other parts of the body. Metered dose inhalers also help drugs work faster (three to six minutes compared with one to three hours for other types of medications).

Even young children (five years and older) can be taught to use a metered dose inhaler. Ask your doctor or nurse to show you and your child how to use one, and be sure the child practices in the doctor's office.

1. Always check to see that the inhaler canister has medication in it. Make note of the doses the child takes and compare to the total number in the canister so you can calculate how much medication is left.

2. Shake the canister well.

3. Have the child stand or sit upright.

4. Instruct the child to open his or her mouth and hold the inhaler one to two inches away. Tell the child not to put the mouthpiece in his or her mouth unless the child is using a spacer. (Note: If the child is using a dry powder inhaler, he or she will need to close lips tightly around the mouthpiece and inhale quickly.)

5. With the child's mouth open, have him or her breathe in slowly (three to five seconds) and, at the same time, press down firmly on the canister to release the medication.

6. Tell the child to hold his or her breath for ten seconds to allow the medicine to reach deep into the lungs.

7. Repeat puffs as directed by your doctor. Wait one minute between puffs to allow the drug to penetrate the lungs better.

Younger children, in particular, will likely have more success using an MDI if they use a spacer, a holding chamber that attaches to the metered dose inhaler. Using a spacer, the child will get less medication in the mouth, on the tongue, and in the air, and more in his or her lungs. A spacer also makes it unnecessary to coordinate breathing with discharging the medication, makes the child less likely to gag or cough on the medication, and can help prevent an oral yeast infection (thrush).

Instruct your child to use the spacer exactly the same way as a metered dose inhaler, except:

• After attaching the spacer to the inhaler according to the manufacturer's directions, instruct your child to shake the canister and press down on the canister in the inhaler. This will deliver one puff of medication into the holding chamber.

• Instruct your child to put the mouthpiece of the spacer into his or her mouth between the teeth and breathe in slowly (for a young child, a face mask can be used). Have the child hold his or her breath for a few seconds and breathe out. Repeat for the prescribed dose.

Teach your child to clean both the metered dose inhaler and the spacer once a day by rinsing them with warm running water. Let them dry completely before reusing. Twice a week, wash the plastic mouthpiece with mild dishwashing soap and warm water. Rinse and let air dry.

How Can a Nebulizer Help My Child?

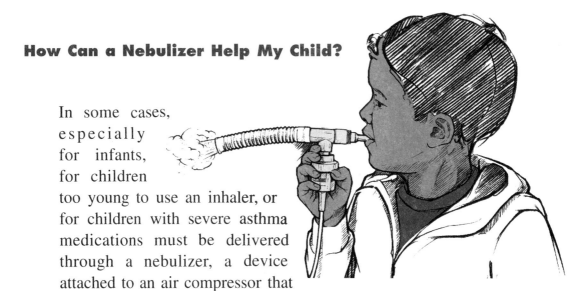

In some cases, especially for infants, for children too young to use an inhaler, or for children with severe asthma medications must be delivered through a nebulizer, a device attached to an air compressor that delivers a fine mist of medicine or saline deep into the lungs.

These devices may be small and hand-held or larger and attached to compressors. They generally consist of a cup, a mouthpiece with a T-shaped mask or mouthpiece, and tubing that connects the device to the air compressor. Your doctor can help you select the right type of equipment for your child. Since each type and brand of nebulizer varies, be sure to get specific operating instructions from the equipment manufacturer.

It's important to use the nebulizer correctly. Always wash your hands before using.

1. Measure the correct amount of saline and place it into the nebulizer cup. Add the correct amount of medication. (It's often easier to use premeasured medications.) Be careful not to touch the inside.

2. Attach the mouthpiece to the T-shaped part and then to the cup (or fasten the mask to the cup).

3. Turn on the compressor and have your child exhale completely.

4. Put the mouthpiece in the child's mouth and have him or her seal the lips around it tightly (or place the mask on your infant's or child's face). Hold the nebulizer straight to obtain the best mist.

5. Tell your child to take slow, deep breaths through the mouth and hold each breath one to two seconds before exhaling. This allows the medication to go deeply into your child's lungs.

6. Have the child continue until all the medicine is used up from the cup (10 to 25 minutes).

7. Store the medication as directed.

You'll need to care for and clean your child's nebulizer properly to ensure it works properly and to prevent serious infection.

1. After each use (or once every day if not used), wash your hands and disassemble washable parts of equipment. (Mask or mouthpiece, T-shaped part, and cup. Tubing should not be washed.) Wash these pieces in warm running water for 30 seconds. (Do not use bleach, vinegar, or very hot water.)

2. Rinse with warm running water and shake off excess water.

3. Place on clean towel and allow to air dry.

4. Reassemble the pieces and connect the device to the air compressor. Run the machine for 10 to 20 seconds to dry the inside of the nebulizer.

5. Disconnect the tubing from the air compressor and store the nebulizer in a clean, dry plastic bag.

6. Once or twice a week, soak the washable parts of the nebulizer in a solution of one part distilled vinegar and two parts distilled water. Toss the solution out after use (don't reuse). Repeat steps 3, 4, and 5.

7. Once or twice a week, wipe the surface of the air compressor with a damp (not soaked), soapy sponge or cloth, or alcohol or disinfectant wipe. (Never put the air compressor in water.) Cover the air compressor with the supplied cover.

8. Replace the nebulizer filter when it appears discolored.

   • Remove the filter cap by turning it counterclockwise.

   • Push the used filter out with a pencil.

   • Insert the new filter into the cap and replace the cap onto machine. (Never try to wash or reuse an old filter.)

What Medications Can Help?

There are two types of asthma medications currently in use: **bronchodilators and anti-inflammatories** (see medication chart on page 52). **Bronchodilators** dilate the airways of the lungs for easier breathing. They relax the smooth muscles that line the breathing tubes, which makes the airways wider and easier to move air through. These medications come in tablets, capsules, liquids, inhalers, injections, and rectal suppositories. If your child has symptoms less than once or twice a week, a bronchodilator medication may be all he or she needs to control the asthma.

Beta$_2$-agonists (or beta-adrenergic agonists) are bronchodilators that relax smooth muscles in the airways and may inhibit the release of certain inflammatory chemicals in special cells called mast cells. These medications may be inhaled using a metered dose inhaler or nebulizer, or inhaled as a powder-filled capsule using a device called a dry powder inhaler. They may also be swallowed as a liquid or tablet or taken as shots. Most often, inhaled beta$_2$-agonists are used as treatment for asthma attacks or to prevent exercise-induced asthma symptoms.

One of the potential problems with inhaled beta$_2$-agonists is that some people overuse them. More frequent use indicates that the asthma is worsening and may require different medications. *If your child is using a beta$_2$-agonist drug every day or more than three or four times in a single day, he or she should see the doctor for a treatment plan reevaluation.*

Your child should take beta$_2$-agonist medication as soon as early warning signs come on. Asthma episodes are easier to stop if the child has taken the medication promptly. If your child needs more medication than the prescribed dosage, talk with the doctor. When your child is also using inhaled cromolyn sodium or inhaled steroid medications (see pages 50 and 51 for further discussion of these drugs), have him or her use the bronchodilator inhaler first to open the airways and increase the effectiveness of these medications. If your child misses a dose, have him or her take it as soon as possible and space the remaining doses for the day at even intervals. Don't double the dose to catch up! Also, watch for and report these and any other side effects to your child's doctor: increased heart rate, palpitations, nervousness, sleeplessness, headache, nausea, vomiting, tremor, shaking feeling.

Theophylline is a mild to moderate methylxanthine bronchodilator (also called xanthine bronchodilator). It comes in three forms to be swallowed: tablets, capsules, or liquid. In severe episodes, it can also be injected directly into the bloodstream. In a sustained-release form, this drug lasts for several hours and is often used for controlling night-time asthma symptoms.

Theophylline works after it reaches a certain level in the blood and must be taken regularly to be effective. It can be used daily without losing its effectiveness and without producing unwanted side effects. However, side effects such as nausea, vomiting, stomachaches, loss of appetite, dizziness, headaches, or irritability can occur if the dosage is too high for your child. The doctor may need to check your child's theophylline blood level regularly to ensure the drug is at the correct dosage.

Instruct your child to swallow (but not chew) theophylline in tablet or capsule form. It should also be taken with food, not on an empty stomach. If your child forgets to take this medication, have your child take the normal dosage as soon as he or she remembers (don't take twice as much). Then talk with the doctor about how to get back on your child's regular schedule. Be sure your child sees the doctor regularly so he or she can monitor theophylline blood level. Let the doctor know if your child experiences these or other side effects: nausea, vomiting, stomach cramps, diarrhea, headaches, muscle cramps, irregular heart beat, and/or feeling shaky or restless.

Anti-inflammatory drugs work to interrupt the inflammatory process and prevent the airways from becoming chronically irritated and swollen. They also decrease the amount of mucus in the lungs and can help to make other drugs work better. This class of drugs includes **oral or inhaled corticosteroids** and **cromolyn sodium** or cromolyn-like drugs. **Steroids** are the most effective anti-inflammatory available and may be taken as a tablet or liquid, or inhaled using a metered dose inhaler. They can also be given as a shot in a doctor's office or emergency room for serious episodes.

Corticosteroids are not the same as the anabolic steroids taken by many weightlifters and other athletes. Many parents are afraid of corticosteroids because they've heard horror stories about long-term side effects. Oral steroids, taken over a long period of time, can cause a wide range of side effects such as cataracts, high blood pressure, bone thinning, weight gain, muscle weakness, and growth slowing in children. However, doctors usually prescribe oral steroids for short periods of time and try to avoid their long-term use. Using oral steroids for a short period of time may cause increased appetite, weight gain, fluid retention, changes in mood, and high blood pressure. However, these minor side effects end when the medication is stopped.

Inhaled corticosteroids act in the same way to control asthma as oral steroids, but they are inhaled directly into the lungs and produce few side effects. Two common side effects with inhaled steroids are a yeast infection of the mouth (thrush) and an irritation of the upper airways, which causes coughing. Both of these problems can be eliminated by using a spacer with the metered dose inhaler and having your child rinse his or her mouth and swallow after taking the medication.

Don't expect inhaled corticosteroids to work right away. It may take as long as one to four weeks for inhaled steroids to be fully effective. Your child should take oral steroids with milk or food (to reduce side effects). Also, make sure your child doesn't stop taking, skip, or decrease his or her steroid medication without talking with the doctor first. Always let any doctor or dentist know if your child is taking a steroid medication, especially if the child is having immunizations, surgery, or emergency treatment, or if the child has a serious infection or injury, or is having dental work done. Report these side effects to the doctor: decreased or blurry vision, fever or sore throat, sore mouth or rash in the mouth or throat, frequent urination, increased thirst, mood changes, signs of infection, or skin rash.

Cromolyn (brand name Intal) is a nonsteroidal anti-inflammatory that prevents the allergic reactions that trigger asthma symptoms. It is used in mild to moderate cases of asthma. Cromolyn is available as an inhaler, as a powder in a capsule for use in a dry powder inhaler called a Spinhaler, or in a liquid for use with a nebulizer. Cromolyn prevents symptoms, but doesn't work once symptoms have started. To be effective, it must be taken every day. It must be taken 5 to 60 minutes before exercise or exposure to other asthma triggers such as animal dander. The effects last for 3 to 4 hours.

Nedocromil (Tilade) is a newer, nonsteroidal anti-inflammatory that is used like Cromolyn. It may be more effective for some people than Cromolyn.

Drugs Frequently Used to Treat Asthma

Medication	Brand Names	How Given
Inhaled Bronchodilators Metaproterenol Albuterol Terbutaline Pirbuterol Ipratroplium	Alupent, Metaprel Proventil, Ventolin Brethaire Maxair Atrovent	Inhaled
Systemic Bronchodilators Theophylline *Adrenergic Medications* Metaproterenol Albuterol Terbutaline	Terbutaline, Theo-Dur, Slo-bid, Aminophylline, Marax, Tedral, others Alupent, Metaprel Proventil, Ventolin, Brethine, Bricanyl	Primarily by mouth By mouth or injection
Inhaled Anti-inflammatory Medications Cromolyn Nedocromil *Inhaled Corticosteroids* Beclomethasone Triamcinolone Flunisolide	 Intal Tilade Vanceril, Beclovent Azmacort AeroBid	 Inhaled Inhaled Inhaled
Systemic Corticosteroid Medications Prednisone Triamcinolone Methylprednisolone Dexamethasone	 Deltasone Aristocort Medrol Decadron, others	By mouth or injection

WORKING WITH SCHOOLS AND OTHER CARE PROFESSIONALS

Children spend a lot of time in school, and teachers and other school officials can play a big role in helping the child manage his or her asthma and live a normal life. It's important that teachers, coaches, and other care providers don't treat the child differently or draw attention to the child by being overcautious or fearful of having to cope with an asthma attack. Reassure school personnel and others who care for your child that he or she has been trained to recognize asthma symptoms and respond immediately with self-care. School personnel also need to know how to recognize early warning signs and be able to respond to both mild and severe symptoms.

How Can I Help School Personnel Respond to My Child's Asthma?

- **Set up a meeting.** Teachers, coaches, and the school nurse should meet with you and/or your partner and be told that your child has asthma and what to do if symptoms develop.

  ➤ Let them know your child's early warning signs.

  ➤ Tell them what to do, including what medications to administer and how quickly they can expect them to work.

  ➤ Give them a list of the medications your child takes, the medication schedule and dosage, and possible side effects.

  ➤ Include telephone numbers of people to contact if your child has breathing problems.

  ➤ List your child's doctor's phone number and address.

- **Encourage the school to make medication easily accessible and as pleasant a routine as possible.** Some schools require that bronchodilators be kept in the nurse's office. Unfortunately, if medications aren't easily available, children may skip doses. See if arrangements can be made to allow your child to keep his or her medications on hand. (This may require a written authorization from your child's doctor.)

- **Encourage teachers and coaches to make the classroom, locker room and gym as "trigger-free" as possible.**

- **Suggest that teachers educate other students about asthma with educational materials or guest speakers.**

- **If your child has severe asthma, consider carrying a beeper so you can be reached quickly.**

- **Provide school personnel with a copy of your child's treatment plan or a letter or other document with pertinent information.**

Asthma First Aid for Educators

The American Lung Association suggests these first aid tips:

- Help the child assume an upright position with shoulders relaxed.

- Talk quietly and reassuringly to the child.

- Encourage the child to take the appropriate medications.

- If medications don't appear to be working, notify the emergency person listed in the child's records.

Signs a Child Needs Immediate Medical Help

- Breathlessness. The child doesn't talk or talks in one- or two-word phrases.

- Child's neck muscles tighten with each inhalation.

- Child breathes rapidly, even at rest.

- Lips and nails are bluish or grayish.

- Chest is retracted (chest skin is sucked in).

Information for Teachers and the School Nurse

_____ has asthma.

Asthma triggers: (in order of frequency)

_____
_____
_____

Signs of asthma episode: (in order of frequency)

_____
_____
_____

Early warning signs:

_____
_____

Medications which need to be taken at school:

Drug_____ Time_____ How often_____
Drug_____ Time_____ How often_____

Exercise restrictions:

_____
_____
_____

Steps to take during asthma episode: (in order of priority)

1._____
2._____
3._____
4._____
5. Contact parent if response to 1-4 is not prompt.

Emergency numbers:

Parent:_____
Physician:_____

MANAGING YOUR CHILD'S ASTHMA AT HOME

In addition to working in partnership with your child's doctor, school officials, and other care providers, there is plenty you can do at home to help manage your child's asthma. This includes:

- **Helping your child assume responsibility for his asthma by identifying and avoiding asthma triggers.**

- **Responding quickly and effectively to asthma warning signs.**

- **Encouraging your child to stay active.**

How Can I Help My Child Identify Asthma Triggers?

As we discussed in previous sections, asthma can be brought on by a wide range of "triggers" such as allergens (pollens, molds, animal dander, foods, or additives), irritants (smoke, sprays, air pollution, strong odors), infections, physical changes (exercise, cold air), and strong emotions. It's vitally important to the management of your child's asthma that you and your child identify as many of these triggers as possible so they can be avoided. While not all asthma episodes can be traced to an identifiable trigger, many of them can.

Your major tool in identifying your child's asthma triggers will be an **asthma diary**. In this notebook, you'll record everything that happens to your child when he or she has asthma symptoms. If your child is older, he or she can do much of this work. Even younger children can become involved in the "detective game" of identifying triggers.

First, list your child's known asthma triggers. Next, begin keeping track of your daily observations. List the date, when the symptoms started, and what your child was doing at the time and in the hours before the symptoms began. Make notes about where your child was and who else was present. Be sure to include what the environment and the weather were like. Then write down what you think might have triggered the symptoms. Even if you're not sure, make a guess.

After several weeks or months, you should begin to see patterns in the diary. Perhaps your child's symptoms are connected to particular places, activities, or weather conditions. It's likely these are some of your child's asthma triggers.

How Can I Help My Child Avoid Asthma Triggers?

Once you know what your child's asthma triggers are, you can take steps to make his or her environment as trigger-free as possible. It's not possible to keep your child away from all his or her asthma triggers, but you can reduce exposure.

- **Rid the environment of dust mites as much as possible.** Dust mites—tiny microscopic creatures that thrive in dust and humidity—are a major cause of allergies and a common asthma trigger. If dust mites are a trigger for your child, it's important to keep your home and especially your child's bedroom as free as possible of places dust mites live.

  ➢ **Go rug-less**. Carpeting catches dust mites. If you must use rugs, use throw rugs that can be washed often. A room with carpet has 40 to 100 times more potential allergens in the air, despite cleaning.

  ➢ **Use chemical agents to kill dust mites in the house**.

  ➢ **Vacuum with a filtered vacuum cleaner.** Put a filter on the exhaust port of your vacuum to keep the dust and dirt from recycling back into your environment. Newer vacuum bags are "dustless" and are able to filter 10 times better than older varieties.

  ➢ **Keep your child from sleeping or lying on overstuffed furniture.** The less over-stuffed furniture you can live with the better.

  ➢ **Enclose your child's mattress and pillow in zippered casings** that don't allow dust in or out.

  ➢ **Switch your child's down or feather pillows** for dacron/polyester fiberfill.

➤ **Use a dehumidifier** if you live in a moist climate. Humidity of less than 50 percent discourages dust mites.

➤ **Don't clean when your child is present.**

• **Eliminate animal dander if your child is allergic to it.** Animal dander—the dead dry skin that flakes off the animal—can also trigger asthma symptoms.

➤ **Go pet-less.** If animal dander is one of your child's allergens, it's probably best not to keep furry or feathered pets. Reptiles and fish are OK.

➤ **Bathe pets often.** If your child is too heartbroken to give up his or her pet, bathe the pet weekly in warm water to control the dander.

➤ **Ban pets from your child's bedroom.** Don't allow your pet in your child's bedroom or on furniture.

➤ **Wash hands frequently.** Teach your child to wash his or her hands immediately after handling any animal.

• **Clean the air.** Allergens in the air such as pollens and molds and irritants such as smoke may trigger your child's asthma symptoms.

➤ **Don't allow smoking in your home.**

➤ **Encourage your child not to smoke or be around secondhand smoke.**

➤ **Control mold in sinks and tubs with bleach.**

➤ **Close windows.** Keep home and car windows closed during peak allergen seasons.

➤ **Install home and auto air conditioning.** An air conditioner can filter out half the pollen in the air, especially if it's set on "recirculate." Be sure the filter is cleaned regularly.

➤ **Talk with a member of your health care team about using a high-efficiency particulate air (HEPA) filter.** These can be rather expensive and are available in medical supply houses.

➤ **Pay attention to the local pollution and pollen counts.** If the pollution or pollen indexes are high, encourage your child to stay indoors with the windows closed.

➣ **Avoid wood-burning stoves.** If your home is wood-heated, consider changing to cleaner-burning electric or gas heat. Avoid kerosene lamps and heaters as well.

- **Help your child avoid respiratory infections.** Viral infections are common triggers among children.

  ➣ **Encourage your child to avoid people who have colds, influenza, or other respiratory infections.**

  ➣ **Make sure your child gets a well-balanced diet, plenty of rest and adequate exercise.**

  ➣ **Have your child's respiratory infections treated promptly by a doctor.** You may want to ask your doctor about annual flu shots for your child.

- **Cut your child's exposure to chemicals.** A surprising number of common household products, hobby chemicals, and personal hygiene products such as deodorant and hair spray can trigger asthma symptoms in many children.

  ➣ **Don't use room deodorizers.**

  ➣ **Adopt nonchemical measures to control weeds and pests in the garden.** For example, use beneficial insects and nematodes to control harmful insects; pull weeds and apply mulches instead of spraying herbicides.

  ➣ **Use nonallergic cleaning products** such as baking soda, lemon oil, mineral oil, club soda (spot remover), mild unscented soaps, and white vinegar.

How Can I Recognize My Child's Asthma Warning Signs?

Children's asthma episodes seldom come without warning. By learning to recognize your child's early warning symptoms and teaching your child how to recognize these signs, you can take quick action and prevent flare-ups.

In addition to the signs listed on page 60, watch how your child is breathing. Is he or she hunched over? Are the child's neck muscles tense? Does the child's nostrils flare when he or she breathes in?

Common Asthma Episode Warning Symptoms

Your child's warning signs will be unique to him or her. Some common signs include:

- Light wheezing
- Drop in peak flow meter reading
- Coughing
- Difficulty breathing
- Rapid breathing
- Restlessness
- Chest tightness
- Fatigue

- Itchy, scratchy, or sore throat
- Sneezing
- Headache
- Fever
- Runny nose
- Dark circles under the eyes
- Itchy or watery eyes
- Nasal and sinus congestion

Asthma warning signs in an infant are more difficult to spot. Because an infant's lungs are less developed, an asthma attack can quickly progress to respiratory failure. Watch for these signs in your baby: less alert and responsive; failure to nurse or feed; chest retracted or hyperinflated; rapid breathing during sleep; softer, shorter cry; or changes in skin color. **These are signs of a medical emergency. Get help fast!**

Responding to My Child's Asthma Warning Signs

Don't wait for symptoms to get worse when you see early warning signs.

- **Stay calm and reassure your child.** Your child's fear can make breathing even more difficult. Encourage the child to breathe slowly through the nose, and to purse the lips and blow out evenly through the mouth.

- **Administer the appropriate medication.** Your child's asthma treatment plan should outline exactly what medicine you should give your child and how much.

- **Have your child assume a comfortable breathing position.** If your child is lying down, prop him or her up with pillows for easier breathing. Or have the child sit up and lean forward slightly on elbows or arms. Make sure there's plenty of fresh air in the room.

- **Obtain a peak flow meter reading.** If your child is five years or older, have the child use the peak flow meter so you can judge the severity of the episode.

- **Don't have the child drink large amounts of liquids or breathe warm, moist air from a shower or vaporizer or re-breathe into a paper bag; and don't give your child over-the-counter medications without the doctor's permission.**

When Should I Call the Doctor?

Your child's asthma may get worse even though you've done all the things outlined in the treatment plan. Call your doctor if any of the following situations occur:

- Your child wheezes, coughs, or has shortness of breath even after medication has had time to work. Most inhaled bronchodilator medications should work within five to ten minutes.

- Your child's peak flow meter reading gets worse or doesn't improve even after using the bronchodilator.

- Your child has chest pain.

- Your child has difficulty breathing (child's chest and/or neck is pulled or sucked in, he or she is hunching over).

- Your child has problems walking or talking.

- Your child stops playing and can't start again.

- Your child's lips or fingernails appear gray or blue. **This is a medical emergency symptom. Get help now!**

- **When you call the doctor or hospital:**

  > **Tell the doctor your name, speaking slowly and clearly.**

  > **Describe your child's symptoms.** Include current and usual best peak flow meter readings if available.

  > **Let the doctor know what medicines you've given the child and when.**

  > **Listen carefully.** Make sure you understand the doctor's instructions.

How Can I Encourage My Child To Stay Active?

Physical activity is important for any child's health and it's particularly important for a child with asthma. In addition to conditioning the heart and lungs, and making them more efficient, participating in physical activities like other children will help your child feel normal. Unfortunately, some children—and some parents—become so fearful that activity will trigger attacks, they avoid sports and other physical activities.

• **Don't place arbitrary restrictions on your child's activities.** Allow your child to explore his or her capabilities through experience.

• **Allow your child to choose his or her own activities.** Talk with your child about which activities he or she feels unable or unwilling to participate in.

• **Give medication in advance, if appropriate.** Exercise is a trigger for some children. If it is for your child, have him or her take medication when preparing to exercise. Also, have your child keep a bronchodilator on hand "just in case."

• **Use a peak flow meter.** Encourage your child to measure his or her lung function before, during and after exercising.

• **Warm up/cool down**. Teach your child to warm up before and cool down after exercising. Also teach him or her to breathe through the nose, which warms, moistens, and filters the air and makes it less irritating to the airways. During cold weather, a scarf or muffler over the nose and mouth will help warm the air.

• **Praise your child.** Give your child positive feedback for participating in physical activities.

• **Get him or her involved in asthma camp.** The American Lung Association sponsors camps for children with asthma that help them expand their range of physical activities as well as better manage their asthma in a supportive environment. Being with other children who have asthma in a camp setting can help your child feel less different and more accepting of his or her condition.

Glossary

allergens—Substances such as animal dander, dust, molds, and pollens that cause allergic reactions in sensitive (allergic) individuals.

anti-inflammatory—Asthma medications that stop the inflammation of the airways that can lead to symptoms.

asthma—An inflammatory disease of the lungs. It is characterized by increased sensitivity of the windpipe and airways to various "triggers" (such as pollen, dust, and cold air) that causes the smaller airways (bronchioles) to narrow and make breathing difficult.

beta$_2$-agonist (or beta-adrenergic)—A type of bronchodilator that opens (dilates) airways.

bronchial tube—Tubes or airways that conduct air in and out of the lungs.

bronchodilator—Asthma medication that relaxes airway muscles, which helps open the airways.

corticosteroid—An anti-inflammatory medication used to treat asthma.

cromolyn sodium—A type of nonsteroidal anti-inflammatory medication used to treat asthma. This drug can be helpful for allergic-type asthma.

episode, flare, or flare-up—A sudden worsening of asthma symptoms.

exercise-induced asthma (or exercise-induced bronchospasm)—Symptoms such as coughing, chest tightness, wheezing, and fatigue triggered by physical activity.

immunotherapy (or desensitization or hyposensitization)— Commonly called allergy shots, this form of therapy involves administering allergens in gradually increasing doses to decrease sensitivity to the substances.

metered dose inhaler (MDI)—A hand-held device that delivers a measured (metered) dose of asthma medication in an aerosol spray or powdered form.

nebulizer (or aerosol therapy)—A device attached to an air compressor that delivers a fine mist of asthma medication or saline (salt water solution) deep into the lungs.

obstruction—Blockage of the airways caused by contraction of bronchial muscles, mucus formation, inflammation, and swelling of the lung tissue.

peak expiratory flow rate (PEFR)—Maximum rate at which air can be expelled, measured in liters per second.

peak flow meter—A hand-held device that measures the force of air exhaled from the lungs. It's commonly used to detect early signs of an asthma episode.

reversibility—Changes in the airways during an asthma episode are not permanent; the airways may return to normal spontaneously or, more commonly, as a result of treatment.

spacer—A holding chamber that attaches to the metered dose inhaler. This device helps deliver more medication to the lungs, decreases gagging and coughing, and can help prevent a yeast infection of the mouth (thrush) when taking inhaled steroids.

spirometer—A device used to measure airway flow.

theophylline—A type of bronchodilator asthma medication.

triggers—Substances, activities, or conditions that cause the airways to react and asthma symptoms to occur.

RESOURCES

There is a wide range of books, directories, organizations, and other resources for families with children who have asthma. This partial list can get you started.

American Lung Association
1740 Broadway
New York, NY 10019-4374
(212) 315-8700

The ALA listed in the white pages of your phone book has more than 300 local chapters. The ALA provides a variety of booklets and pamphlets about asthma, including "Facts About Asthma," "What Everyone Needs to Know About Asthma," "Facts About Peak Flow Meters," "Childhood Asthma: A Matter of Control," and "The Asthma Handbook." In addition, they have special publications just for children, including "The Best of Super Stuff: For Kids with Asthma" and "Let's Talk About Asthma: A Guide for Teens." Also, ask about the ALA asthma camps for children.

National Asthma and Allergy Network/Mothers of Asthmatics
3554 Chain Bridge Rd. Ste. 200
Fairfax, VA 22030
(800) 878-4403 or (703) 385-4403

This nonprofit group provides support for the parents of children with asthma. It publishes the MA Report, a newsletter, and TeamWork, an annual resource list of publications, organizations, and product vendors, and sponsors asthma camps.

American Academy of Pediatrics
Box 927
141 NW Point Blvd.
Elk Grove Village, IL 60009-0927
(708) 228-5005

Write for the comic teaching book "Captain Wonderlung: Breathing Exercises for Asthmatic Children." Available in English, Spanish and French.

American Academy of Allergy and Immunology
85 West Algonquin Ste. 550
Arrington Hts. IL 6005
(800)842-7777 or (708) 427-1200/1400

This group provides pamphlets on asthma, allergies, mold and pollen.

**Asthma and Allergy Foundation of America/
Mothers of Asthmatics, Inc.**
1125 15th St. NW Ste. 502
Washington, DC 20005
(800) 727-8462 or (202) 466-7643

Local chapters throughout the country offer support groups, school programs, community workshops, and conferences on asthma and allergies.

National Heart, Lung, and Blood Institute
31 Center Dr. MSC 2480
Bethesda, MD 20892-2480
(301) 496-4236

The institute provides free publications on recognizing early signs of asthma, identifying and controlling triggers, managing asthma attacks, taking medications properly, and coping skills. Some of its titles include "Asthma Reading and Resource List," "Living with Asthma," "Open Airways," "Air Power," and "Air Wise."

National Jewish Center for Immunology and Respiratory Disease
1400 Jackson St.
Denver, CO 80206
(800) 222-LUNG

This nationally recognized treatment center provides information about asthma and other lung diseases via a toll-free line.

National Asthma Education Program
NHLBI Information Center
P.O. Box 30105
Bethesda, MD 20824
(301) 251-1222

This organization provides free copies of the "NHLBI Asthma Reading and Resource List" and the "Resource List for Asthma Education in Schools."